PALEO
DIET

WORLD CLASS RECIPES, TOP
INGREDIENTS, AND LIVING HEALTHY

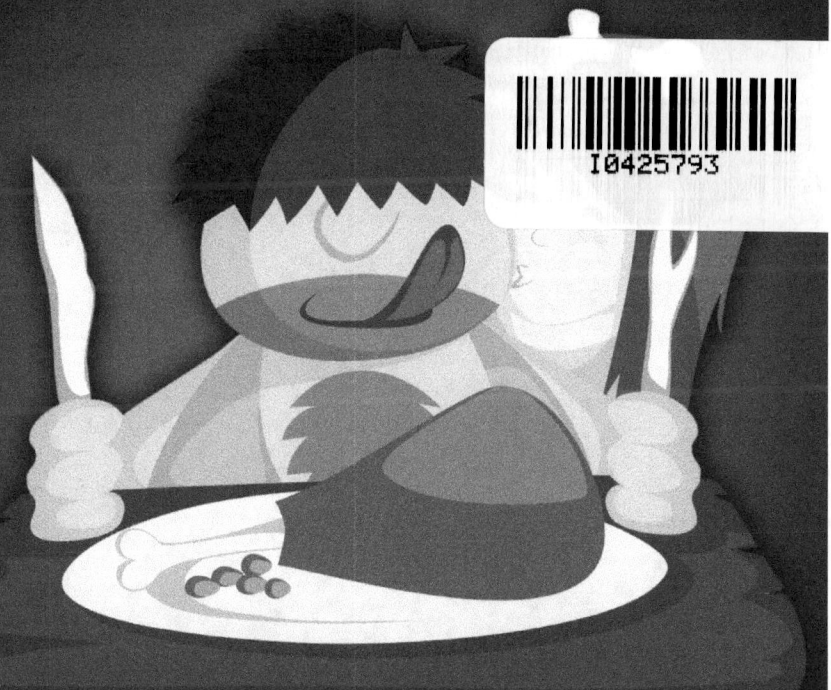

DAN THOMPSON

PALEO DIET

- ❖ World Class recipes
- ❖ Top ingredients
- ❖ Living healthy

PREFACE

The bane of this century is processed food, transfats, and saccharides. Obesity, cancer, heart disease, Alzheimer's, ADHD in children, and so many other ailments are plaguing humanity today. To counter the ill effects of the present age, a variety of diets are in vogue. This book is going to take an in-depth look at a trending new age diet – *The Paleo Diet.*

The Paleo Diet is believed to be the diet followed by our ancestors in the Stone Age. It primarily consists of meat, fish, fruits, berries, and tubers, sans the dairy products, cereals and the processed food.

It was Dr. Boyd Eaton's paper "Paleolithic Nutrition: A Consideration of its Nature and Current Implications" that brought to the fore the health implications of this caveman diet to modern society. I have referred to stalwarts like Dr. Loren Cordain, who has contributed significantly in the field of evolution and diet. This book will attempt to give you an understanding of following a food plan that ensures that your body is not ingesting and digesting food that is laden with carcinogenic additives and preservatives.

This book attempts to provide a brief introduction to Paleo diet before plunging into the strengths of the various Paleo ingredients. In the course of the book you will be surprised to find that several delectable dishes can be made from Paleo ingredients.

I will also briefly touch on how exercise and Paleo diet can go hand in hand and how muscle building is so possible when following this caveman diet.

Hopefully, on this journey you can become an ardent Paleo follower and progress towards a fitter, healthier and happier you.

INDEX

Chapter 1 - What is Paleo Diet?

Chapter 2 –Health benefits of Paleo Diet

Chapter 3 –Exercise on Paleo Diet

Chapter 4 – Scrumptious Recipes

Chapter 5 – Staying Motivated

WHAT IS PALEO DIET

Origins

Our bodies were not designed to digest refined and processed food overloaded with additives and preservatives. We are simple machines who need simple food. In prehistoric times, humans ate whatever was available or whatever they could hunt.

It is a well-known fact that ancient humans lived long, healthy lives. Obesity, heart disease, cancer, and other lifestyle diseases so prevalent in the modern day were unknown during those times. Prehistoric humans were known to be lean, agile and had a muscular build. It definitely was their lifestyle and the diet they followed that contributed significantly to their health.

It was Dr. Boyd's paper in the New England Journal of Medicine that showcased to the world the correlation between the Paleolithic way of eating and a healthy life. It was further propagated by Dr.Loren Cordain who has authored the internationally acclaimed book, The *Paleo Diet*.

He can in fact be considered the *Guru* of Paleo diet. He is a well-known expert on Stone Age diet and its positive effect on human health.

What is a Healthy Diet?

For a healthy body our nutrition chart should consist of carbohydrates, fats, proteins and essential vitamins, and minerals.

Carbohydrates consist of starches, sugars, and fibers. To keep diabetes and obesity at bay one should opt for low glycemic index foods in comparison to starches like rice and white potatoes.

Moving on to fats, you should know that there are good fats and bad fats. Good fats are the mono saturated fats, polyunsaturated and omega-3 fatty acids, while the bad fats are trans fats and saturated fats. To maintain the health of the heart and keep the levels of triglycerides and cholesterol in the healthy range, you should avoid the bad fats and intake more of the good fats.

Proteins are the most important part of your diet. Every single cell requires protein to function. Proteins are required for muscle health, tissue repair and for hormone and enzyme functioning.

Finally vitamins and minerals as we all know are required for leading a healthy, deficiency-free life. They keep the body on the right track.

What is Paleo Diet?

Now that we know what is considered a normal diet, we need to see if the Paleo diet meets all the requirements.

Prehistoric humans were nomads and roamed place to place. The only weapons they had were very crude and carved out of wood. They had access to the fruits on the trees, the roots and tubers down below, the fish in the water and the occasional game they hunted down. They survived primarily on roots, tubers, berries, fruits, vegetables, meat, and fish. Their diet was bereft of all kinds of dairy products, whole grains, legumes, and sugars. Alcohol and coffee were unknown to them. Fortunately, they were not exposed to the ills of adulterated, refined, sugary foods that seem to be destroying the very core of our health system today.

As you can see, a strict Paleo diet has a low glycemic index, is rich in proteins – which not only improve the musculature of the body, but also help in weight loss – has healthy fats like mono saturated fats and Omega 3 fats that are crucial for the overall wellbeing of the heart, the lipid profile and regular brain functions; is loaded with vitamins, minerals, and phytochemicals that are known to possess many disease fighting abilities. A Paleo diet is also low in sodium and carbs while being high in potassium.

Let's turn our attention the Paleo ingredients now.

Paleo ingredients

Before we proceed further we need to understand that many of our ingredients might not be exactly the same as the cavemen used; hence we will settle for the next best things available and try to stay as true as possible to the original ingredients. For example, it is not possible to go hunt your next meal or sadly even fish because of the several cases of mercury poisoning in fish is alarming and it is best to obtain fish from a farm or from known fishmongers where you know the quality of the fish.

With proper understanding of what comprises a true Paleo diet you can formulate a diet plan. Remember to keep your menu simple to be a true follower of a Paleo diet.

Given below is the entire group of food that is considered Paleo.
- Meat and fish
- Vegetables
- Fruits
- Nuts and seeds
- Oils and fats

Meat and Fish

The prehistoric caveman could easily hunt his meal and he had no need to preserve it with preservatives. Since it is not possible to hunt your meat and fish your best bet would be to eat organic meat whenever possible. Listed below is the meat which is considered to be Paleo.

Buffalo meat: The meat from buffalos is leaner when compared to beef, and since this meat is less popular the chances of it been hormone injected is rare.

Lamb: A less popular meat choice but all the same it is a Paleo ingredient.

Pork: In the Stone Age, this was most likely wild boar, but pork and related pig products are good substitutes.

Poultry

Poultry plays a significant role in our diet plan on a day to day basis.

Turkey: You will be happy to know that on Christmas you can have your turkey. It is Paleo.

Chicken: The age old question of what came first- the hen or the chicken suffices to say, the chicken must have been around even in the Paleolithic age and hence chicken wings, legs, thighs and the chicken as a whole is considered Paleo; actually it is a staple for Paleo adherents.

Eggs: One of the most nutritious food substances available ever, eggs are a great source of protein. Ensure that you eat organic and free-range eggs.

Seafood

Fish comprised a main part of the Paleolithic diet. Most fish are rich in protein and omega 3.

Bass: A rich source of omega 3 and protein, the bass must have been one of the main ingredients of the Paleolithic diet

Halibut: Not only is it rich in omega 3, it is also rich in vitamins and minerals.

Mackerel: Another fish known to have several health benefits like lowering cholesterol, combating cancer, and boosting immunity.

Sardines: A great source of vitamin D along with proteins

The other common fish which you might consider are Clams, Lobster, Salmon, Shrimp, Swordfish, Tilapia, Trout, and Tuna.

Veggies

The Paleo diet is rich in vegetables which were easily grown and could be eaten raw. Most of the vegetables are rich sources of fiber and phytonutrients that are so essential to health. Here below I have covered the A-Z of all vegetables that complement the meat and the fish thus rendering a meal complete. Most of the vegetables can be grilled, steamed or eaten raw.

- Artichoke, Asparagus
- Beets, Broccoli, Brussels Sprouts
- Cucumber ,Cabbage, cauliflower, Carrots, Celery, Collard Greens
- Eggplant, Endive
- Green Onions
- Kale
- Mushrooms, Mustard Greens
- Onions make a great veggie for Paleo followers because they are easily available and can be used to enhance the flavor of any dish.
- Parsley, Parsnip, Peppers, Pumpkin
- Radish, Rhubarb, Romaine, Rutabaga
- Seaweed, Spinach, Squash, Swiss Chard
- Tomato, Turnips
- Watercress
- Zucchini

Fruits

Be it a Paleo diet or a regular diet, fruits are an essential part of a balanced diet. In a Paleo diet, however, fruits are one of the main sources of carbs. All fruits are rich in vitamins, fiber and minerals. They are also loaded with sugars, so care should be taken that they are eaten in moderation and never in juice form.

- Apple, Apricot, Avocado
- Banana, Blackberries, Blueberries, Boysenberries
- Cantaloupe, Cherries, Cranberries

- Cherimoya– a wonderful fruit filled with vitamin B6 and vitamin C it is rich in fiber and protein.
- Figs
- Grapefruit, Grapes, Guava
- Honeydew
- Kiwi
- Lemon, Lime, Lychee
- Mango
- Orange
- Papaya
- Passion Fruit:an excellent addition to any kind of diet because it has both iron and vitamin C in it. Vitamin C is necessary to absorb iron.
- Peaches, Pears, Persimmon, Pineapple, Plums, Pomegranate
- Raspberries
- Star Fruit, Strawberries
- Tangerine
- Watermelon

Nuts and Seeds

The Paleo diet is such an all-encompassing diet that none of the good things are missed. The goodness of nuts and seeds, which are the richest sources of mono saturated fats, can't be undermined in the Paleo diet. They not only contribute to the good fats but are also helpful in building muscle and adding extra calories for those who want to build muscle.
- Almonds
- Cashews
- Hazelnuts
- Macadamia Nuts
- Pine Nuts, Pumpkin Seeds
- Sunflower Seeds: An essential part of any Paleo diet, it is high in Vitamin E, which is not available easily in the Paleo diet otherwise.
- Walnuts

Nut oils

Since modern day cooking is not possible without any oil at all unlike our ancestors, the use of oils derived from nuts and seeds are considered Paleo.

Avocado Oil –It is believed to lower blood cholesterol, prevent cancer and also contribute to healthy hair and skin. It is predominantly used as a salad oil.

Butter – Yes, that's right. Though it is a dairy product and so not Paleo, the allowance here is that butter made from grass fed cows can be had on a Paleo diet. Clarified butter popularly known as ghee can also be used to enhance the taste of your meals.

Coconut Oil – It is a good-for-all oil which can be used not only for cooking, but also to treat cuts, bruises, allergies and dry skin. Use the extra virgin, organic oil.

Macadamia Nut Oil -They are extremely beneficial in lowering the triglyceride levels, improving the immunity system, promote bone health and improve energy levels. In addition to that they prevent several chronic diseases while improving the gut health.

Olive Oil – It is well known that this oil helps prevent cancer, keep the risk of diabetes low, prevents stroke, takes care of the heart and fights osteoporosis.

From this extensive list of ingredients it is clear that a Paleo diet cannot be tasteless and hard to follow. As a matter of fact with some ingenuity you can be Paleo at every single meal of the day. The only difference will be that you will be eating healthier, fresher food with no additional preservatives and additives that ruin your health.

HEALTH BENEFITS OF PALEO DIET

Healthy living is a combination of a disciplined life, which comprises of a balanced diet, regular exercise and rest. When you adhere to a healthy lifestyle you can be assured that several diseases are shown the door.

The critics of Paleo diet will argue themselves hoarse that a diet which is shorn of dairy, legumes, and grains cannot be beneficial especially for hard core athletes and those who are looking to build muscles; they require more carbohydrates than the rest. It is difficult to meet the glycogen demand of their muscles from the carbs derived from fruits and vegetables. It is wearisome, but not impossible to work with a Paleo diet and yet perform HIT without feeling the lack of energy.

Let me list out a few benefits of the Paleo diet to show you that the diet really works.

Benefits of Paleo diet

1. The Omega 3 fatty acids present in Paleo diet play a prominent role in brain functioning and in helping normal growth and development. It is also beneficial for brain health and that of the heart and eyes too.They are known to reduce inflammation and reduce the risk of cardio vascular diseases, cancer and arthritis
2. All the animal protein helps in muscle building and reduction of fat.
3. Sugary foods and junk food that you eat put a huge amount of stress on your digestive system. By eliminating the bad from your diet you are automatically improving your gut health.
4. By eating free range eggs and pasture raised meats, you are ensuring that you don't eat hormone induced food which is linked to several cancers. And to top it, the free range eggs are three times more rich in omega 3 fatty acids when compared to normal eggs.

5. Vegetable are rich in nutrients and vitamins and the wonderful phytochemicals which have anti-aging properties besides other benefits.
6. Loose fat: with processed food out of the way and a low carb diet you are automatically on the way to losing weight. Not only the unnecessary carbs but the fat which follows these carbs is also kept away.
7. With Paleo diet you will not need another energy drink ever again. Why? Because all low glycemic index foods release energy slowly thus making up for the lack of energy which normally results with intake of sugary substances.
8. Paleo diet will improve your BP; your glucose tolerance decreases, your insulin secretion and your insulin sensitivity increases. The lipid profile too shows marked improvement. In fact, this is one of the reasons that people who are suffering from any medical condition can try this diet, because natural food never harms.
9. Everyone acknowledges that the modern western diet is the cause for many of the major diseases prevalent today. By substituting an unhealthy diet with vegetables, fruits and animal fats, the risk is reduced substantially.

Cons of Paleo diet

There is no such thing as a perfect diet in the world. Everything has pros and cons and it is upto us to decide if the pros outweigh the cons.
1. The amount of carbs that you get from vegetables and fruits is not sufficient for the athlete and the sportsman. To meet their energy needs, athletes who follow a Paleo diet need to get their carbs from white potatoes. The absence of these in a Paleo diet hinders their progress.
2. Vegetarians will not be able to follow this diet because they cannot eat both important sources of protein namely meat and legumes.

3. It can be confusing as to what comprises Paleo and what is not; and hence sticking to the diet becomes a bigger challenge.

Thus you can see that the drawbacks are minimal and can be easily countered with a few adjustments to the diet. The road is uphill no doubt, but it is not impossible to reach the peak.

Cost of Turning Paleo

At the outset, trying to adhere to this diet might seem expensive because of the insistence on organic, free-range food that is void of preservatives. But take a closer look, and you will realize that in the long run you will be saving several hundred dollars that you would otherwise spend on health care and treatment.

Secondly, to save on big money, buy your ingredients in bulk and preserve them. Oils can be bought and stored in the pantry for long. Try to get your meat directly from the farmer, that way you can be sure of the quality of the meat too. It can be frozen for future use. Similarly, buying whole fish from your fishmonger is a better option than buying from the frozen section of a supermarket.

Finally, vegetables and fruits too can be bought in bulk. Buy sufficient quantity in season and preserve them naturally by lacto fermentation or freezing.

Even though it seems like opting for a Paleo diet might be expensive, you will be glad for the change because the long-term benefits far outweigh the costs you incur initially. Add to this the money you will save on expensive treatments, it is the obvious choice. Moreover, with proper planning you save instantly on your purchases.

Muscle building and Paleo diet

Before the end of this chapter we should to put to rest once and for all the issue of body building on Paleo diet. It is possible to build muscles staying on a Paleo diet. By increasing the dose of nuts and seeds in your diet you will increase the calorie content and also the good fats needed for muscle building. This along with appropriate exercises will definitely take you to your goal.

EXERCISE AND PALEO

Any exercise must be fun and appealing. If you do the same routine every single day, you tend to get bored and your muscles get used to it, which means you need to exercise for longer to get the same benefits. Variations in exercise and workout regimes are the best way to get the most out of your routine.

Regular exercise as you know improves your immunity, reduce the risk of heart diseases, diabetes, blood pressure, osteoporosis, and stroke; thereby enriching your life and also prolonging your life. In the stress prone environs of today it is paramount that everyone exercise regularly.

Exercise not only has health benefits, it also makes you look good, which boosts your self-confidence to take on the world.

Any kind of physical exercise requires lot of energy, stamina and endurance. While the exercises themselves will help in building endurance and stamina, it is the diet which provides the necessary energy and also the nutrition required thereafter to repair the tissues and cells which are affected during an exercise.

Now comes the all-important question – Can an athlete survive on a Paleo diet alone?

Before we analyse whether a pure Paleo diet can be productive for a full-time sportsperson, let's take a look at some Paleolithic forms of exercises

Paleolithic exercises

- **Walking**
  Our ancestors walked long distances; today we needn't walk to reach places but we must walk to stay healthy. Simple brisk walking which can be varied by either hiking sometimes or backpacking ensures that all sets of muscles are exercised.

- **Swimming**
  Once again, the Stone Age man had no access to or hadn't the knowledge to build boats or rafts. They swam to cross the rivers and other water bodies, thereby doing mild cardio.

- **Lifting heavy objects**
  The Paleolithic man would have lifted rocks, pushed boulders and trees out of the way.

- **Sprinting**
  Cardio all the way it is. At regular intervals sprinting brings in loads of benefits.

Thus, to embrace the "Paleo factor" while exercising, you can try all the aforementioned activities, along with some modern exercises like pushups and pull ups and dips. The reps and variations will bring in variety, keep boredom out of the picture and exercise all muscles.

You must have noticed that cardio is not part of the Paleo exercise routine. You should avoid it for the simple reason that it requires high carb diets which will only detriment your progress in the long run. And it goes without saying that the Paleolithic humans never subject themselves to intense cardio, at least on a daily basis. The only time they were in the fight or flight mode was when they were being chased by wild animals!

Having said that, a true blue athlete who wants to follow Paleo and stick to his rigorous regime need not be disappointed. First and foremost the inclusion of animal fat and fish in the diet along with low GI carbs mean that you are on the way to building your muscles and losing the unnecessary fat from your system.

For the high carb requirement when on a Paleo diet increase the intake of fruits like pineapple and bananas and cherries which are very high on carbohydrate. With time your body will get used to the carb reserves in the body and work accordingly so you get the best results.

The ground rule for every exercise is the important rest and recovery period. Do not miss out on this crucial post-activity phase because this is when your tissues repair themselves.

You don't need high intensity exercises to stay fit; Paleo exercises coupled with Paleo diet and good rest will do the trick. But for professional athletes, and those keen on pushing themselves, it is essential to tweak the diet a bit and consume the occasional high carb to prevent severe muscle damage in the long run.

SCRUMPTIOUS RECIPES

All the talk about exercise must have got your taste buds tingling and waiting for some yummy food. But you are on a Paleo diet and any kind of diet means tasteless food right? Wrong! I have listed below some exciting recipes to prove that Paleo can be healthy and tasty at the same time. You will be surprised to find that Paleo recipes are not only delicious but also easy and light on the stomach, all without the addition of artificial food enhancers. Wow!

Banana Bread

How is bread possible without flour? There are several substitutes for the normal flour in the Paleo world. Here I have used coconut flour. A warm banana bread is a great way to start the day - drizzle some honey atop the warm moist bread and enjoy it.

Ingredients
- mashed ripe bananas- 4
- eggs- 4
- almond butter- 1/2 cup
- Ghee- 4 tbsp.
- coconut flour- ½ cup
- Cinnamon- 1 tbsp.
- baking powder- 1 tsp
- baking soda – 1 tsp
- salt- ¼ tsp

Method
1. Using a blender or a whisk combine the banana, the eggs, almond butter, ghee nicely. Preheat oven to 350 degrees F and line a loaf tin with parchment paper.
2. Combine the flour and the rest of the ingredients to the above mixture. Once well mixed transfer the same to the loaf pan

and bake for 50-60 minutes or until a toothpick inserted into the center comes out clean. Cool the bread before slicing it.

Roasted Butternut Squash Soup

Butternut squash is a rich source of folates, riboflavin, niacin, vitamin B-6, thiamin and pantothenic acid. Not only is the very essential B complex present but also minerals like zinc, iron, calcium, and potassium and phosphorous are also present in the vegetable. It is free of any saturated fats and cholesterol, and often finds a place on diets for weight loss.

Ingredients
- Butternut squash – 1 (about 5 lbs.)
- green apple, sliced and cored - 1
- small yellow onion, finely diced - 1
- carrots, finely chopped- 2
- Olive oil -3 tbsp.
- Cinnamon – tsp.
- Salt- to taste
- Cumin- ½ tsp(optional)
- chili powder – 1 tsp(optional)
- chicken broth or water – 3 cups

Method:
1. Preheat oven to 400 degrees F. In a large bowl mix the squash along with olive oil, cinnamon, salt, and cumin. Combine it well enough to coat the squash completely. Distribute it evenly on a baking sheet.
2. Now you can mix the carrots and apples and onions in the same bowl and transfer them to another baking tray lined with a baking sheet. Roast for 35-40 minutes until soft, stirring once.
3. The next step is to boil the roasted veggies along with the broth or water and some salt and chili powder. Simmer covered for 20 minutes.
4. Puree and serve warm. Garnish with fresh mint for a little zing.

Paleo Nachos

Yep, nachos can be Paleo too. What better snack than Paleo nachos to munch on and watch Sunday night sports?

We make chips of sweet potatoes which are the healthy carbs as they have a low glycemic index. They are also a good source of fiber, potassium, vitamins - especially Vitamin A and beta carotene. They are a low sodium vegetable.

So the nacho dish is Paleo all the way as it has a low GI carb topped with protein rich spicy meat, vitamin rich tomatoes and guacamole. A recipe which will definitely replace your regular nachos anytime; even the Paleo critic will have to agree.

Ingredients
- medium tomatoes, diced and seeded - 2
- fresh cilantro, finely chopped- 2
- Lime juice- 2 tbsp.
- guacamole- 2 cups
- Green onions, finely chopped – 2 tbsp.

Chips
- large sweet potatoes -3
- Melted coconut oil- 3 tbsp.
- salt- 1 tsp

Meat topping
- medium onion, finely diced - 1
- Coconut oil – 1 tbsp.
- green chili, diced - 1
- Ground beef - 1lb.
- cloves garlic, minced - 2
- smoked paprika- 1/2
- ground cumin – ½ tsp
- Tomato paste- 1 tbsp.
- Canned diced tomatoes -12 oz.

- salt- to taste
- Pepper- ½ tsp (optional)

Method

1. **Sweet potato chips**: Preheat the oven to 375°F. Peel the potatoes and slice them very thinly. Next mix them with the coconut oil and salt and place them on a baking sheet and in the oven for 10 minutes. Flip the chips and bake for another 10 minutes. Just keep a watch in the last few minutes and remove chips as they start browning.

2. **Meat Topping:** In a skillet heat the oil and sauté the onion and chili for 3-4 minutes, stirring continuously so as to not burn the onions. Once they are nicely done, add the beef and cook for another 5 minutes. This is followed by adding the garlic, tomatoes, tomato paste and the rest of the spices. Mix it well and bring the mixture to a boil and then simmer on medium flame before cooking it covered for 20-25 minutes. Remember to stir frequently.

3. Once the beef mixture is done, add the chopped tomatoes and lime juice and garnish with cilantro. Check if salt is okay and bring down from the flame.

4. Now is the best part; assembly. Arrange the sweet potato chips on a platter and cover it with the beef mixture. Put the guacamole on the top of the mixture and garnish with the green onions.

The Paleo nachos are a perfect and light snack that taste excellent without adding on high calorie sauces and dips.

Grilled Vegetable Salad

Salads need not be always boring and dull. We invariably enhance the salad with dressing them up with mayonnaise if nothing else. Can mayonnaise be Paleo? Anything is possible. Make your own mayonnaise at home using 2 egg yolks, 3 tsp lemon and ½ cup olive oil. In a blender blend the yolk and 1 tsp lemon juice. Slowly add the oil to form an emulsion and once the mayonnaise thickens add the rest of the lemon juice. Voila, Paleo mayonnaise is ready. It's that simple!

Ingredients

- medium zucchini 3
- medium yellow squash 1
- red bell pepper 1
- yellow bell pepper 1
- red onion, thinly sliced 1
- Asparagus ends trimmed1 lb.
- Extra virgin olive oil, for drizzling

For the sauce

- 1/4 cup Paleo mayonnaise -1/4 cup
- Juice of 1 lime
- cloves garlic, crushed 2
- Cumin 1 tsp
- Salt & pepper, to taste

Method

1. Slice the vegetable to any shape of your choice and drizzle salt and pepper on top of the slices. Preheat the grill and place the vegetables on it. Coat the veggies lightly with oil. You have to grill for 10-12 minutes before serving.
2. In another bowl whisk the ingredients of the sauce together and season with cumin.
3. Serve the veggies along with the sauce or just gently mix the sauce with the grilled veggies.
4. It makes a nice accompaniment to the soup.

Paleo Mojito

A refreshing drink alongside a great meal is always welcome and if it is a mojito without the alcohol and the sugar what else would you need?

Ingredients

- Strawberries 10

- juice of 1 lime
- mint sprigs 2
- ice cubes 10
- Honey 1 tbsp.
- sparkling water

Method
1. Roughly blend the strawberries and the mint springs. Add lime juice and honey to the mixture and mix it well.
2. Place the ice cubes and the mixture in a glass and top it with sparkling water.
3. Paleo mojito is ready to be sipped and enjoyed.

Frittata

Can there be a frittata which is dairy free and gluten free and yet taste delicious? Well the recipe below will surprise you. It can be a breakfast option or a snack or can even be a dinner option.

Ingredients
- Coconut oil 1 tbsp.
- finely chopped red pepper ½ cup
- finely diced onion 1/3 cup
- crispy bacon, 3 slices
- chopped kale, de-stemmed and rinsed 2 cups
- Eggs 8
- almond or coconut milk ½ cup
- Salt and pepper to taste

Method
1. Preheat oven to 350 degrees F. Whisk the eggs and milk together. Season with salt and pepper. Keep it aside for the time being.
2. Heat a skillet and add the coconut oil. Once the oil is hot, sauté the pepper and onion until soft. Add kale and cook till it wilts. This whole process takes about 5 minutes.

3. To the above mixture add the bacon and the eggs and cook till the frittata sets.
4. Put this frittata in the preheated oven and cook for 10-15 minutes or until it is fully cooked. Take it out. Slice it and serve.

Paleo Desserts

No Flour No Sugar Paleo Brownie

A perfect dessert for the sweet toothed person. These mouthwatering fudgy brownies are so good that you can't stop with one. And the best part is that there is no flour, butter or sugar. Can a dessert get healthier than this? It is simple and easy to make.

Ingredients
- Almond butter1 cup
- maple syrup 1/3 cup
- egg 1
- Ghee 2 tbsp.
- vanilla 1 tsp
- cocoa powder 1/3 cup
- baking soda ½ tsp

Method
1. Preheat the oven to 325°F. In a large bowl, whisk together the almond butter, maple syrup, egg, ghee, and vanilla. Stir in the cocoa powder and baking soda.
2. Pour the batter into a 9-inch baking pan. Bake for 20-23 minutes, until the brownie is done, but still soft in the middle.

Paleo Dark Chocolate Mousse

The name itself brings a smile on the face. It is the perfect dessert to follow a perfect Paleo meal.

Ingredients

- 1 ripe avocado
- 1/4 cup date paste
- 1 tbsp. unpasteurized honey
- 1 cup full fat coconut milk
- 1/2 cup organic cacao powder
- 1 tsp instant coffee
- 1/4 tsp Ancho Chili powder
- 1/4 tsp Himalayan salt
- 1 tbsp. pure vanilla extract

Method

1. Puree the dates paste, avocado, honey and coconut milk until it turns into a smooth paste.
2. To this puree add the cacao powder, coffee, chili powder, salt and vanilla and continue to blend till all the powders are nicely incorporated into the mixture.
3. Next whisk this entire mixture into a fluffy consistency either using a hand whisk or a stand mixer.
4. Your chocolate mousse is ready to be refrigerated. Transfer the mousse to individual bowls and refrigerate for 4-6 hours at least.
5. Though this mousse can be had straight away the taste is enhanced when had cold.

The above recipes will help you host your friends and family to a Paleo day wherein you can start with the breakfast and end with the dessert – all Paleo. They will sure be surprised with the palatability and the great taste of Paleo food.

Staying Motivated

It feels great to read about the benefits of Paleo diet and even better to know that you can exercise and still stay on Paleo, and best to know that some amazing desserts and meals can be prepared with Paleo ingredients. Wonderful, right? Unfortunately staying on course in a new diet is by far the biggest challenge that anyone faces. It is not easy to break old habits and patterns of eating; the devil is waiting to pounce at the first instance of weakness and drag you back to the hell of unhealthy eating habits.

It is said, "With great power comes great responsibility." I will tweak it around and say with great responsibility great power comes - the power of healthy living, the power of long lasting energy, the power which comes with a fit body and the power which comes with a razor sharp brain.

You have decided to adopt the Paleo diet; that is a great responsibility. Staying on any kind of diet is not easy, especially when benefits are not instantaneous. It is so easy to fall back on unhealthy routines and lose shape and then get into a self-pity mode and start a vicious circle that doesn't end.

The craving for junk food can be difficult to control and only the bravest and the most disciplined manage to adhere to a diet.

How to Stay Motivated

I have listed below a few guidelines which if followed diligently will definitely ensure that you stay on track and stick to your Paleo diet.

Maintain a daily food log
It is a very good habit to write down everything that you eat and drink. Your journal should contain all details of the food and the quantity they were taken in. You can always go through the log and

stay motivated to see that you have been sticking to your diet plan, or you will be able to see that you are falling and will make effort to get back on track immediately.

You are responsible for following your diet and your journal will be a faithful companion in this journey.

Find support

Things become a lot easier when you have the support of family and friends. Convince a friend or a family member to try the diet out with you. It is always fun to share your little victories and minor slips with someone who will understand. You can support and motivate each other to stay on track.

Download an app

Your smart phone is your best friend. The entire world is present in that rectangular piece of technology; utilize it to stay on track. The app will aid you stay on track and also you can interact with other members of the same community and learn new ways and methods to prevent you from slipping.

Experiment in the kitchen

Since much of Paleo cooking is fresh and preservative free, you have to cook from scratch. In the process, try to experiment with various combinations and arrive at new recipes and dishes that you can relish with your family.

Meal planning

Make a list of all the meals of the day and for the week. Note it down in your journal. Jot down the basics of the recipes too, thus you will be prepared all the time and won't be able to slip back into bad eating habits for lack of preparation or easy availability of healthy food.

Surround yourself with positive quotes

Words have great power. Keep positive workout quotes on your phone, on your refrigerator, in your bathroom, on the TV, in your smart phone - essentially everywhere. The constant reminder will keep the spirit alive in you and will help you in maintaining your resolve to follow the diet.

Juggle the dishes
Variety is the spice of life; so too with food. Juggle your breakfast and lunch recipes to boost your nutrition and improve your digestion.

It is not easy to stay motivated and adhere to a diet. You will slip and fall several times, but as long as you pick yourself up each time with a greater resolve to achieve better health you are good to go. Then there will critics who will try to influence you and also convince you about the futility of the diet; these are hurdles you have to cross before you reach your goal of perfect health.

Empower yourself with health and happiness and a better you are just around the corner.

CONCLUSION

The Paleo diet is here to stay. On a daily basis following a Paleo diet is not too much; you just need to be prepared. Empty your pantry of all the junk and processed food. Stock your ladder and your fridge with fruits and vegetables and other Paleo ingredients.

The Paleo diet will benefit your heart, cholesterol level, lipid profile, thyroid health in addition to helping in weight reduction and rendering you a good physique. Any diet followed prudently alongside sufficient exercise and rest will yield results.

To achieve the best results from your diet you have to understand your body and work with it and not against it. Combine HIT with low intensity cardio while avoiding chronic cardio. For the professional athlete, some minor modifications in the diet can be made to incorporate carbohydrates to meet the body's demand for higher energy. The Paleo diet will definitely enrich your life. Try it and I can assure you, there will never be a moment of regret.

www.ingramcontent.com/pod-product-compliance
Lightning Source LLC
Chambersburg PA
CBHW072022290526
45787CB00013B/1759